# Instant Pot

## *Instant Pot Pressure Cooker Cookbook With Easy And Healthy Recipes*

**LELA GIBSON**

LELA GIBSON

# **CONTENTS**

# Introduction

I want to thank you and congratulate you for buying the book, "Instant Pot: Instant Pot Pressure Cooker Cookbook With Easy And Healthy Recipes".

This book has lots of finger licking Instant Pot recipes guaranteed to make you enjoy your every meal.

These days, life is becoming a lot busier than it ever was. The situation is so bad that we hardly have the time to prepare home cooked meals that we can enjoy. In such cases, opting for take outs is the norm.

In addition to being costly to live on takeouts, it is also highly likely that the foods many of us buy on our way home from work, over lunch, or in the morning on our way to work are unhealthy and likely to put us on the path to having different health complications. The good news is that people are increasingly becoming creative in developing different products meant to make life manageable even in the midst of all the 'busyness'.

One such product if the Instant Pot. Designed with the ability to act as a slow cooker, pressure cooker, rice cooker, skillet and a host of other kitchen appliances, the instant pot can truly transform your cooking positively. The only challenge that you might have when you have newly acquired an Instant Pot is the shortage of recipes that you can make. Worry not though because this book has lots of delicious recipes that will certainly transform the way you cook your breakfasts, lunches, and dinners. By reading this book and taking action, you can bet that you will no longer have excuses why you cannot have fresh, home cooked meals every single day.

Thanks again for buying this book. I hope you enjoy it!

Assuming that you understand what an instant pot is and how to use it well (e.g. releasing pressure using quick release method or natural release method) and how to care for the Instant Pot, we will start by discussing delicious breakfast recipes using an instant pot.

# Section 1: Breakfast Recipes

## 1: Instant-Pot Breakfast Cobbler

**Serves: 2**

**Ingredients**

2 tablespoons of sunflower seeds

¼ cup (30 g) of pecan pieces

¼ cup of shredded coconut, unsweetened

½ teaspoon of cinnamon, ground

3 tablespoon of coconut oil

2 tablespoon of local honey

1 plum, diced

1 apple, diced

1 pear, diced

Coconut whipped cream, optional

## Directions

Place the cut fruit into the Instant's pot bowl and then spoon in the coconut oil, honey, and season with cinnamon.

Lock the lid in place and press the Steam function. The time will automatically be set to 10 minutes.

Now cook the fruits until done and then quick release pressure. Carefully remove the lid and use a slotted spoon to move the cooked fruit into a serving bowl.

At this point, put sunflower seeds, pecans, coconut into the liquid left in the cooking pot and press the sauté button. Let the mixture cook while shifting them occasionally.

As soon as the contents appear well browned and toasted, remove from the pot and top with the fruits. Serve warm and garnish with whipped cream if you like.

## 2: Breakfast Porridge in the Instant Pot

*Serves: 2*

## Ingredients

1 tablespoon of Maple Syrup or Honey

2 teaspoon of Coconut Oil, melted

1 cup of Water

1/2 cup of Dried Coconut Shreds, Unsweetened

1/2 cup of Pecan Halves

1/4 cup of Pepitas, shelled

1/2 cup of Cashews (raw, unsalted)

Coconut sugar, ghee or fresh fruit, garnish

## Directions

Place the ingredients, apart from maple syrup, coconut oil and water, in a food processor or blender.

Puree until the mixture achieves an almond-like consistency; this should take about 30 seconds.

Pour the mixture into the Instant Pot and stir in maple syrup, oil, and water. Lock the lid and press the Porridge function.

Set the timer to 3 minutes, allow the porridge to cook, and then quick release pressure and stir the porridge.

Serve the porridge topped with ghee, coconut sugar, or fresh fruit.

### 3: Breakfast Quinoa

**_Serves: 6_**

## Ingredients

¼ teaspoon of cinnamon, ground

½ teaspoon of vanilla

2 tablespoons of maple syrup

2 ¼ cups of water

1 ½ cups of quinoa, uncooked

Pinch of salt

Toppings: sliced almonds, fresh berries and milk

## Directions

In the cooking pot of an Instant Pot, add cinnamon, vanilla, maple syrup, water, quinoa, and salt.

Set the timer to 1 minute and cook the ingredients at high pressure.

Natural release the pressure for about 10 minutes then quick release.

Carefully open the lid then fluff the quinoa. Serve the dish with sliced almonds, berries and milk if you like.

## 4: Cranberry Steel Cut Oats

## Serves: 6

## Ingredients

2 teaspoon of vanilla

½ teaspoon of salt

¼ cups of maple syrup

½ teaspoon of nutmeg

1-2 teaspoon of cinnamon

1 teaspoon of fresh lemon juice

2-4 tablespoons butter and/or virgin coconut oil

1 ½ cups of fresh cranberry

4 apples, diced

3 cups of water

1 cup of yogurt

2 cups of milk

2 cups of steel cut oats

## Directions

Start by using butter or coconut oil to grease the bottom of the Instant pot container.

Soak all the ingredients (apart from the maple syrup, vanilla, and salt) in the Instant Pot overnight.

Come morning, add in the salt and syrup and start cooking the porridge.

Allow the Instant Pot to get to pressure in around 20 minutes and then start cooking. Once done, open the valve to allow quick release of pressure.

Now stir in the vanilla and serve using the milk.

## 5: Oatmeal Apple Crisp

## Serves: 2

## Ingredients

2 ½ cups of water

1/3 cup of melted margarine

½ teaspoon of salt

1 teaspoon of cinnamon

½ cup of brown sugar

1/3 cup of flour

1 cup of quick cooking oats

1 tablespoon of lemon juice

4 cups of apples, peeled and sliced

## Directions

Sprinkle the lemon juice on the apples and then combine the oats, salt, margarine, brown sugar, flour, and cinnamon.

Arrange alternating layers of the oat and apple mixture inside a buttered metallic bowl that will fit in a pressure cooker and then use aluminum foil to cover the bowl.

In the pressure cooker, place water and position the metallic bowl on a rack inside the cooker, secure the lid, and place the pressure regulator on a vent pipe

Cook for about 20 minutes while the pressure regulator rocks slowly and then cool and serve.

## 6: Steel Cut Oats

*Serves: 2-3*

## Ingredients

Dash of salt

1 tablespoon of oil, preferably extra virgin olive oil

2 cups of water

½ cup of Steel Cut Oats

## Directions

In the instant pot, combine the above ingredients and then cook for 10 minutes at high pressure.

Once done, natural release the pressure and then do a quick release. Let the valve drop and then open the lid.

Stir the oats and allow to rest for a minute in order to absorb water.

Now top with the milk, granola or chopped nuts, as well as fresh or dried fruits such as strawberries or blueberries.

You can add any sweetener you prefer such as agave syrup, maple syrup, brown sugar, or honey.

## 7: Potato-Bacon Hash Browns

***Serves: 4***

## Ingredients

225 g crumbled bacon

2 tablespoons parsley, chopped

1 kg sweet potatoes, washed and peeled

2 tablespoons olive oil

Pepper, freshly ground

Salt

## Directions

1. Process or grate the sweet potatoes in a food processor. Using a strainer, rinse the potatoes by letting them sit under running water for 30 seconds.

2. Using paper towels dry the potatoes, thoroughly, as this helps get crispier hash.

3. Heat oil in a pressure cooker and then add the potatoes, season with salt and pepper then sauté for 5-6 minutes until brown.

4. Add in parsley and bacon. Mix well and then press the bacon and potato down firmly using a wide spatula.

5. Lock the lid and cook for 6-7 minutes under low pressure. Turn off the cooker and quick release.

4. Serve it hot with scrambled eggs, toast, fresh fruit juice or coffee.

## 8: Mini Frittatas

***Serves: 6***

### Ingredients

5 eggs

Desired mix in's: veggies, cheese, meats, the options are endless!

Spices such as salt and pepper

Splash of milk (I use almond milk)

### Directions

In a dish, mix the milk, mix in's and eggs.

Pour the mixture into baking molds. Pour a cup of water into the instant pot, and then place the molds on the rack of the instant pot.

Set the pot to manual high pressure for 5 minutes and once the timer goes off do a quick release.

Serve and enjoy!

# Section 2: Lunch Recipes

## 9: Butternut Squash Pasta

*Serves: 6*

## Ingredients

3 cups of fresh spinach, rough chopped

Salt and pepper to taste

3.5 cups of homemade bone broth

1 pound of penne pasta

½ medium butternut squash cut into 1 inch pieces

1 tablespoon of bacon grease

1 tablespoon of butter

2 cloves of garlic, chopped

1 small onion, chopped

2 tablespoons of olive oil

6 slices of bacon, chopped

Freshly grated Parmesan cheese (optional)

## Directions

Press the Browning or Sauté function on your Instant Pot and allow to heat.

To the cooking pot, add bacon and sauté until crisp. Then remove the bacon from cooking pot and drain it. Reserve the cooking grease.

Now add in oil along with the onions and sauté until the onions cook through.

Add in garlic, sauté for a minute, and then add the pepper, salt, butter, pasta, bacon grease, bacon, and the squashes.

Lock the lid in place and set the timer for 4 minutes. Cook on high pressure until beep sounds then quick release pressure.

Carefully open the lid and add in spinach to the cooking pot.

Serve with cheese if you like.

# 10: Texas Beef Chili

***Serves: 4***

## Ingredients

1 teaspoon of garlic powder

1 teaspoon of paprika

4 teaspoons of chili powder

1 tablespoon of Worcestershire sauce

1 tablespoon of fresh parsley, chopped

1 teaspoon of onion powder

1 teaspoon of sea salt

½ teaspoon of ground black pepper

26 oz. of finely chopped tomatoes

4 large carrots, chopped small

1 large onion, diced

1 green bell pepper, seeded and diced

1 lb. of grass-fed organic beef

Pinch of cumin

Sliced jalapenos, optional

Diced onions, optional

Dairy-free sour cream, optional

## Directions

Activate the Sauté setting, add ground beef to the Instant Pot and cook until brown.

Add the rest of the ingredients and mix well. Cover, lock the lid, and cook on Meat/Stew function for 35 minutes.

Once cooked, quick release or natural release pressure and serve.

## 11: Instant Pot Carne Guisada

***Serves: 4***

## Ingredients

1 tablespoon of potato starch

½ cup of tomato sauce

1 cup of beef broth or chicken stock

½ teaspoon oregano

½ teaspoon chipotle powder

½ teaspoon pepper

1 teaspoon of salt

1 teaspoon of paprika

1 teaspoon of chili powder

1 teaspoon of ground cumin

1 bay leaf

1 Serrano pepper, minced

1 tablespoon of minced garlic

1 onion, diced

1 pound of beef stew meat

2 tablespoons of avocado oil

## Directions

Press the sauté function on your instant pot and then add oil into the Instant Pot. Add in the beef cubes and sear the meat on all sides.

Once the beef cubes have browned, add in the spices, bay leaf, Serrano pepper, garlic and onion. Stir fry for around 2-3 minutes.

Pour in tomato sauce and beef broth and lock the lid. Press on the Meat/stew function and cook the meat for 35 minutes.

Natural release pressure for 10-15 minutes then unlock the lid. Ladle a little of the liquid in a bowl and add in potato flour. Combine and stir the thicker into the pot.

Serve the dish over tortilla or cauli-rice.

# 12: Pork Belly & Spiced "Rice" One Pot

*Serves: 4*

## Ingredients

½ teaspoon of salt

1 tablespoon cumin

1 tablespoon oregano

1 teaspoon turmeric

1 tablespoon animal fat

3 cloves garlic, sliced

1 tablespoon lime juice

2 green onions, sliced

½ cup of cilantro, divided

½ red onion, sliced

½ cup of bone broth

4 cups of riced cauliflower

1 pound of pork belly, cooked and cubed

## Directions

Place all ingredients (apart from cilantro) in an Instant Pot.

Lock the lid and set the timer to 15 minutes.

Cook under high pressure then turn off the cooker. Natural release pressure for about 10 minutes then open the lid and serve.

# 13: Pressure-Cooker Lamb Stew

## *Serves: 4-5*

## Ingredients

¼-½ teaspoon of salt

3 tablespoon of broth or water

6 cloves garlic, sliced

1 bay leaf

1 sprig rosemary

1 large yellow onion

3 large carrots

1 acorn squash

2 lbs. of lamb stew meat, cut into 1″ cubes

## Directions

Prepare the acorn squash by peeling, seeding, and cubing it. You can microwave for a minute before cutting it.

Slice the carrots, peel the onion, and slice it into half moons. Cut the veggies either bigger or smaller as per your choice.

Place all the ingredients into the Instant Pot and cook for 35 minutes at high pressure.

Quick release pressure and unlock the lid. Serve and enjoy.

## 14: Cilantro Lime Rice

***Serves: 6***

## Ingredients

3 tablespoon of fresh cilantro, chopped

1 tablespoon of lime juice, fresh

1 teaspoon of salt

2 tablespoons of vegetable oil

1¼ cups of water

1 cup of long grain white rice

## Directions

In the pot of the pressure cooker, add in rice, a tablespoon of oil and the water, stir well lock the  lid in place, and cook under high pressure for 3 minutes.

Once done, turn off the pressure cooker and natural release pressure in 7 minutes.

Follow this with a quick release and then use a fork to fluff the rice.

Now mix together a tablespoon of oil, lime juice and chopped cilantro into a medium bowl.

Add the rice and toss together to mix all ingredients completely.

## 15: Instant Pot Kalua Pork

***Serves: 8-10***

## Ingredients

1/2 cup water

1 tablespoon liquid smoke

1 teaspoon fish sauce

1/2 cup diced pineapple

1 teaspoon sea salt

1 tablespoon lard or bacon fat

4-5 pound pork shoulder

## Directions

1. Press the sauté button and wait until your Instant Pot displays "HOT". Cut the pork into two pieces, and add lard to the cooking pot.

2. Sear each half of the pork shoulder for 2-3 minutes on each side. Once well browned, remove from the cooking pot and turn off the cooker.

3. Sprinkle salt on the meat, and add in fish sauce, pineapple, water and liquid smoke. Also include other juices from the platter and secure the lid.

4. Press the Manual button and set the timer to 90 minutes. Once the timer beeps, release the pressure naturally.

5. Remove the pork from the cooking pot and transfer the juices into a jar. Using two forks pull the meat apart to remove any excess fat.

6. Remove the fat from atop of the jar and discard. If desired, add some of the juices to the pork.

## 16: Instant Pot shredded chicken

### *Serves: 8*

## Ingredients

1 -2 stalks green onion, green part chopped finely and the white part cut into 1.5 inch pieces

10 dried Chinese red chili

8 - 10 (about 2 pounds) chicken drumsticks

3 garlic cloves, minced

1 (10g) slice ginger, chopped roughly

1 tablespoon peanut oil

Optional: 1 tablespoon (15ml) honey

### *Sauce:*

2 tablespoons Chinese black vinegar or distilled white vinegar

¼ cup dark soy sauce

¼ cup sugar

1 teaspoon sesame oil

2 tablespoons Shaoxing wine

2 tablespoons cornstarch mixed in 2 tablespoons water

***Serve:***

Optional: Hoisin sauce

16-20 pieces lettuce

## Directions

Press the sauté button and pour in one tablespoon of peanut oil.

Toss in the minced garlic, chopped ginger, 10 dried Chinese red chili and the white part of your green onions and ncook slowly until fragrant (this will take about 3 minutes).

Add the chicken drumsticks and sauce mixture into the cooker and close the lid.

Cook at high pressure setting for 12 minutes and allow 12 minutes of natural release.

When done, release any remaining pressure and then carefully pop open the lid.

Take out the chicken drumsticks and place them in a large mixing bowl. Use a fork to shred the chicken and remove all the bones (you can also remove the skin if desired).

For the sauce, remove the Chinese red chili from the cooker, and then press sauté on your instant pot to get the sauce boiling again.

Taste your sauce and add in about 1 tablespoon of honey if you desire to sweeten it.

Mix together the cornstarch and the water and pour this mixture into your sauce a third at a time as you stir until desired thickness is achieved.

Put the shredded chicken back into your now ready sauce and combine.

To serve: Put the pulled chicken on top of lettuce leaves and garnish with the finely chopped green onion. You can also serve the chicken wrap with some Hoisin sauce.

Enjoy!

# Section 3: Dinner Recipes

**17: Pressure Cooker Pot Roast & Gravy**

*Serves: 4-6*

**Ingredients**

6 cloves of garlic, peeled

4 carrots, peeled or scrubbed

2 parsnips, peeled

4 three inch sprigs thyme

1 3-inch sprig of rosemary

2 teaspoons of fish sauce

2 tablespoons of balsamic vinegar

1½ cups of beef broth

Black pepper, freshly ground

A good pinch of salt

4 pounds of chuck roast cut into 4 pieces

Parsley, chopped

## Directions

First season the meat with salt and pepper and put it in an Instant Pot.

Put the rest of the ingredients in the cooking pot, lock the lid in place, and set the timer to 1 hour.

Cook under high pressure then natural release for about 15 minutes.

Remove the roast from the pot and set on a plate. Discard the thyme and rosemary stems.

Pour the liquid from the Instant Pot into a measuring cup or a large jar. When the fat rises to the pot, use a small ladle or large spoon to remove it.

Pour the rest of the liquid into a blander that has veggies and puree until smooth. If need be, season the mixture with salt and pepper.

Using two forks, shred the meat and pour gravy on it. Alternatively, you can stir gravy into the roast.

Serve the roast with mashed or roasted potatoes, cauliflower mash or other roasted or mashed root veggie.

## 18: Beef Stew with Turnips and Carrots

*Serves: 4*

## Ingredients

¼ cup of fresh parsley, chopped

¼ cup of coconut aminos

1 pound of carrots, 1 inch pieces

1 pound of turnips, 1 inch pieces

1 cup of bone broth

1 cup of dry red wine

1 teaspoon of dried thyme

2 tablespoons of cassava flour

1 medium red onion, chopped

2 tablespoons of bacon grease or coconut oil

Salt

1 pound of beef stew meat cut 1 inch pieces

## Directions

Use the sauté function to Preheat the Instant pot and in it, melt 1 tablespoon of fat.

Add seasoned beef, brown on all sides for around 8 minutes; remove the meat from Instant Pot and set aside.

Add the rest of the onions and fat into the Instant Pot and while stirring, cook for 5 minutes or until soft.

Stir in the thyme and cassava flour, cook for 1 minute, and then whisk in wine and scrap browned bits from the bottom of the cooking pot.

At this point, stir in the coconut aminos, carrots, turnips, and broth along with the reserved broth.

Close the lid and press on the Meat/Stew function. Cook then natural release pressure for 10 minutes.

Quick release, open the lid and serve the stew into bowls. Garnish with parsley.

## 19: Maple Smoked Brisket

*Serves: 6*

### Ingredients

3 fresh thyme sprigs

1 tablespoon of liquid smoke

2 cups of bone broth or stock

½ teaspoon of smoked paprika

1 teaspoon of onion powder

1 teaspoon of mustard powder

1 teaspoon of black pepper

2 teaspoon of smoked sea salt

2 tablespoon of maple or coconut sugar

1.5 lb. of beef brisket

## Directions

Remove frozen brisket from the fridge 30 minutes earlier, pat it dry with paper towels, and set it aside.

Prepare the spice blend by mixing together paprika, onion powder, mustard powder, pepper, smoked sea salt, and maple sugar. Season the meat on all sides.

Press the sauté button on the Instant Pot and preheat for 2-3 minutes. Coat the bottom of the cooking pan with cooking oil and add in the meat.

Brown the brisket on all sides until deeply golden. Then turn it—fatty side up—and add thyme, liquid smoke, and the broth. Scrape off any browned bits off the bottom and lock the lid.

Set the timer to 50 minutes then cook under high pressure. Natural release pressure and then remove it to a plate to cool while covered with foil.

Press the sauté button on the Instant Pot to thicken the sauce with lid off for around 10 minutes.

Finally, slice the brisket and serve it with whipped veggie of choice. Drizzle with the sauce and enjoy.

## 20: Stuffed Acorn Squash

***Serves: 3-4***

## Ingredients

½ cup of Parmesan cheese, freshly grated

2 acorn squash, sliced in half

3¾ cup of chicken stock

1 teaspoon of fresh thyme, finely chopped

1 teaspoon of fresh sage, finely chopped

1 teaspoon of fresh rosemary, finely chopped

½ cup of quinoa

1 cup of brown rice

2 garlic cloves, minced

1 teaspoon of salt

1 cup of diced onion

1 tablespoon of butter

Parmesan cheese for garnish

## Directions

Preheat your Instant Pot and then add in butter.

Once melted, add in onion and season with salt. Sauté the onion for 2 minutes

Add in garlic and sauté the ingredients for 1 minute. Add in chicken stock, thyme, sage, rosemary, quinoa, and rice. Stir to incorporate.

In a heat-proof steamer basket, put the acorn squash halves (the cut side up) and position on the trivet.

Drop the steamer basket into the Instant Pot on top of rice with the trivet. Lock the lid and set the timer for 6 minutes.

Cook until done and then quick release pressure. Carefully remove the lid and remove the steamer basket using pot holder or two towels.

Drain excess liquid and set aside the squashes.

Into the rice mixture, stir in Parmesan cheese and let the mixture sit for 5 minutes or until it thickens.

At this point, spoon the rice mixture into the cavity of individual squash half. Top or garnish with Parmesan cheese.

## 21: Instant Pot Vegetarian Chili

*Serves: 4-6*

## Ingredients

½ cup of beer or water

1 cup of frozen corn

1 sweet potato, peeled and chopped

1 14.5 oz. can of diced tomatoes with chiles

1 15 oz. can of Kidney Beans

1 15 oz. can of Pinto beans

1 15 oz. can of black beans, drained and rinsed

¼ teaspoon of cayenne pepper

1 teaspoon of sea salt

1 teaspoon of paprika

2 teaspoon of cumin

1 tablespoon of chili powder

1 jalapeno, diced and seeds removed

1 large poblano pepper, chopped

1 small white onion, chopped

2 cloves garlic, crushed

1 tablespoon of olive oil

## Directions

Press on the Sauté function then preheat the Instant Pot for 1-2 minutes. Add in olive oil to grease the cooking pot.

Add in peppers, garlic, onions, and stir. Sauté until the vegetables are soft (in about 3 minutes).

Toss in salt and other seasonings of your choosing and mix to well coat the veggies. Sauté the vegetables for around 1 minute.

Add in corn, sweet potatoes, tomatoes with juice, beans, and beer or water. Lock the lid in place.

Set the timer to 4 minutes, cook at high pressure, and then quick release; carefully open the lid and stir.

If you need a thicker sauce, Sauté on high for another 3-5 minutes.

Season with extra salt and serve with preferred toppings.

## 22: Potato Salad

*Serves: 6*

## Ingredients

1 teaspoon of cider vinegar

1 teaspoon of yellow mustard

½ cup of mayonnaise

1 tablespoon of chopped fresh dill

3 hard-boiled eggs, chopped

Salt and pepper to taste

1 stalk of celery, chopped

¼ cup of chopped onion

1 cup of water

6 medium red potatoes, scrubbed

## Directions

Put the potatoes in an Instant Pot containing water then cook for about 3-4 minutes at high pressure.

Natural release pressure for 3 minutes, then quick release any remaining pressure, and  open the pressure cooker.

When potatoes are cool enough, peel and dice them.

In a large bowl, alternate layers of onion, celery and potatoes and season each layer with pepper and salt.

Add in the chopped eggs to top up and now sprinkle with dill.

Mix the mustard, cider vinegar, and mayonnaise in a bowl and then fold the mayonnaise mixture gently into the potatoes.

At this point, allow to cool for about an hour before serving the salad.

## 23: Whole Chicken in an Instant Pot

### *Serves: 6-8*

### Ingredients

1 tablespoon of coconut oil

1 cup of water

Seasonings of choice

1 whole chicken

### Directions

In an instant pot, add a cup of water and then place a steam rack inside the cooking pot.

Heat oil in a large skillet and then cover the chicken with various seasonings.

Place the chicken in oil and let the skin sear for 60 seconds on each side; once seared, position it in the steam rack of the cooking pot.

Now lock the lid and set the cooker to "Chicken" setting and cook the chicken for about 20 minutes. To calculate cooking time, allocate 6 minutes for each pound of the chicken.

Leave chicken in the pot for at most 30 minutes then release pressure naturally for 15 minutes.

## 24: Cornish Hens

### *Serves: 2*

## Ingredients

1 1/2 cups water

2 teaspoons Worcestershire sauce, soy free

2 stalks celery, chopped

2 bay leaves

4 cloves garlic, chopped

2 onions chopped

Salt and pepper

2 tablespoons oil

2 Cornish hens

## Directions

1. In an Instant Pot add the oil, and then the hens.

2. Use pepper and salt to season the chicken and then pour the remaining ingredients over the chicken.

3. Seal the cooker and heat under low heat for 8 minutes ensuring the pressure regulator rocks slowly.

4. Remove the contents from the heat and allow the pressure to drop naturally.

## 25: Pina Colada Chicken

***Serves: 4***

## Ingredients

2 tablespoons coconut aminos

1/8 teaspoon salt

1 teaspoon cinnamon

1/2 cup coconut cream, full fat

1 cup pineapple chunks, fresh or frozen

2 pounds chicken thighs cut into 1" pieces

1/2 cup green onion, chopped

## Directions

1. Put the ingredients apart from the chopped onions into a pressure cooker.

2. Close and seal the lid then set to Poultry setting.

3. Cook for about 15 minutes at high pressure. Once cooked turn off the cooker and allow natural release of pressure for 10 minutes.

4. After the valve drops, gently open the lid and remove from the pot. Stir and add a teaspoon of arrowroot starch and tablespoon of water to thicken the sauce.

5. Press the sauté button and continue to cook until you achieve desired thickness.

6. Finally turn off the Instant Pot. Serve the chicken and garnish with green onion.

7. If you like, prepare a coconut cream by chilling a can of full-fat coconut milk in the refrigerator overnight. Later open the can and drain the coconut water.

## 26: Barbecue Pork Spare Ribs

***Serves: 4***

## Ingredients

1/8 teaspoon celery seed

1 teaspoon prepared mustard

1 teaspoon Worcestershire sauce, soy free

5 teaspoons white vinegar

3 tablespoons ketchup

3 teaspoons canola oil

240 ml water

1 teaspoon paprika

1 teaspoon pepper

1 teaspoon onion salt

900 g boneless pork ribs, sliced

## Directions

1. Begin by cutting the boneless pork ribs into small pieces, and then season with paprika, pepper and salt.

2. Heat oil in the pressure cooker and brown the ribs on all sides. Then drain the ribs and put them back into the cooker.

3. Add in the rest of the ingredients and pour them over the meat. At this point, lock the lid and cook the dish for around 15 minutes.

5. Once the time elapses, naturally pressure release and then serve when hot.

## 27: French Dip Sandwich

*Serves: 6*

## Ingredients

1 loaf of Paleo bread

1½ cups of beef stock

2 teaspoons of onion powder

1 tablespoon of minced garlic

1 tablespoon of Worcestershire sauce

1 teaspoon of pepper, freshly ground

1½ teaspoons of salt

6 pounds of chuck roast

## Directions

In an Instant Pot, put beef stock, onion powder, garlic, sauce, pepper and salt, and set the timer to 1 hour if meat is thawed and 1½ hours if frozen.

Cook under high pressure until the meat cooks through.

Separate the meat and juices by passing the mixture through a mesh strainer over a pot. Put the meat in a bowl and use forks to shred it.

Bring the juice to a boil, and then simmer until the juices have reduced by half. Skim off any fat that rise to the top.

At this point, season with salt, and pepper, and then cut the bread into sandwich sizes and split down its center.

Put the shredded meat onto the bread and top with provolone cheese. Put on a cookie sheet and melt the provolone under a broiler until bubbly.

Finally, assemble the sandwich and ladle the sauce in container to make a dip. Serve the sandwich and enjoy.

## 28: Pork vindaloo

*Serves: 6*

## Ingredients

Salt and pepper

3 pounds boneless pork butt roast

1 teaspoon sugar

8 garlic cloves, minced

1 (14.5 ounce) can diced tomatoes

1/4 cup all-purpose flour

1 tablespoon mustard seeds

1 cup low-sodium chicken broth

1 teaspoon ground cumin

1/8 teaspoon ground cloves

1/4 cup minced fresh cilantro

3 onions chopped finely, trimmed and cut into 1-inch pieces

2 tablespoons red wine vinegar

1 tablespoon paprika

2 tablespoons vegetable oil

1/4 teaspoon cayenne pepper

## Directions

Pat dry the pork with paper towels then season it with some pepper and salt.

Press the sauté function on your instant pot, and then add a tablespoon of oil into the cooker pot.

Add half of your meat in and let it cook for about 8 minutes until all sides are nicely browned then transfer to a bowl.

Heat the remainder of the oil in the empty cooker pot until shimmering.

Toss in the onions and ¼ teaspoon of salt and let it cook for about 5 minutes until softened.

Throw in the mustard seeds, cumin, cloves, garlic, paprika and cayenne, stir and let cook for about 30 seconds until fragrant.

Add in the flour, stir and let it cook for a minute. Add the broth and whisk as you smoothen out any lumps and scrape up any browned bits.

Add in the tomatoes, sugar, vinegar, the browned pork together with its juices and the rest of the pork.

Lock the cooker in place and let it cook at high pressure for 30 minutes.

Once done, allow the pressure to release naturally for 15 minutes.

For any remaining pressure, quick release it and remove the lid carefully with the steam escaping away from you.

Before you serve, use a large spoon to scoop away the excess fat from the surface of the soup and stir in the cilantro.

Season with some pepper and salt, serve and enjoy!

# Section 4: Snack Recipes

## 29: Corn on the Cob

*Serves: 3*

### Ingredients

6 ears of corn

### Directions

Break the ears of corn in half and lay in the cooking pot. Stagger the corn to help steam pass through them.

Add about 1 cup of water and securely lock the lid.

Cook on manual for 8 minutes then quick release the pressure. Ensure the corn does not touch the water.

## 30: Re-fried Beans in the Instant Pot

*Serves: 4*

## Ingredients

3 cups of vegetable broth or water

Cilantro

½ cup of salsa

½ teaspoon of black pepper

1 teaspoon of cumin

1 teaspoon of chili powder

1 teaspoon of paprika

1 teaspoon of salt

1 jalapeno, seeded

4 cloves of garlic, peeled and roughly chopped

1 large onion, cut into fourths

2 cups of dried pinto beans, not soaked

## Directions

In an instant pot, add all the ingredients and stir well. Then close the lid and turn the stream valve to a setting of "Sealed"

Select "Manual" setting and then set the timer to 28 minutes. Once cooking is done, allow natural pressure release for 10 minutes.

Open the lid and stir thoroughly. At this point, use a blender or a potato smasher to blend the beans into the preferred consistency.

Once the beans get thick, drain the water off and continue to blend or smash.

Serve the fried beans warm or freeze into portion-sized containers.

## 31: Soy Sauce Eggs

***Serves: 4-8***

## Ingredients

4-8 boiled extra-large eggs

1½ cup Chinese master stock

## Directions

If using a pre-made Chinese master stock, put it into the Instant Pot, secure the lid, and cook for 10 minutes at high pressure.

Quick release and carefully open the lid. Pour the stock into a bowl and allow to cool.

Put a steamer basket into the Instant Pot, add a cup of cold water, and then put the eggs in the steamer basket.

Lock the lid in place and cook for 5 minutes at low pressure if using soft-boiled eggs and 14 minutes if using hard-boiled eggs.

Carefully open the lid and place the eggs in an ice bath for about 5 minutes. Carefully remove the egg shells.

At this point, put the eggs into a warm medium bowl of Chinese stock. Put a paper towel on the eggs and soak into the stock.

As soon as the bowl with Stock and eggs has cooled off, cover and transfer in the fridge for a minimum of 2 hours. A longer duration of time will help the eggs soak more Chinese stock flavors.

Finally, serve the eggs either warm or cold. To warm, simply heat the eggs and stock in a saucepan on medium low heat.

## 32: Southern Style Boiled Peanuts

***Serves: 4***

### Ingredients

Water

¼-½ cup of Sea Salt

1 pound of Jumbo Raw Peanuts

### For Cajun Flavor

Jalapeno Peppers

Fresh Garlic

1 tablespoon of Cajun seasoning

### For Barbecue Flavor

1 teaspoon of Sugar

1 tablespoon of Barbecue Seasoning

### Directions

First rinse the peanuts with cold water. Place the peanuts into the Instant Pot along with salt and cover with water.

Put a trivet or a plate on top to hold the peanuts. Secure the lid in place and cook for 1-2 hours on high pressure.

After the beep sounds, naturally release pressure and let the contents cool for 30 minutes. In case the peanuts are too hard, cook for a little longer.

# 33: Lentils with Chorizo Sausage

## *Serves: 2*

## Ingredients

Pinch of salt

1 bay leaf

½ teaspoon paprika

¾ liter of cold water

4 garlic cloves

1 medium onion

1 large carrot

100g of chorizo sausage

225g of brown lentils

## Directions

Place the lentils, onion, peeled carrot, garlic cloves in the pressure cooker and add vegetables as well as the bay leaves.

Chop the chorizo to about 4 pieces and put in the cooker followed by cold water, paprika, and salt to taste.

Bring the contents to a boil and then cover and lock the Instant Pot. Let the ingredients cook for about 8 minutes.

Once done, turn off, natural release pressure, carefully open the lid, and then discard the bay leaves.

Meanwhile, put carrots, garlic, and onions into the receptacle of a hand blender and puree to desired consistency.

At this point, return the pureed vegetables to lentils, and mix the contents well before serving.

## 34: Steamed Carrot Flowers

### *Serves: 4*

### Ingredients

1 cup water

1 lb. thick carrots, peeled

### Directions

1. Using potato peeler, remove unwanted skin from carrots. Make 4-5 grooves along the stem then cut the carrots into flowers or "coins".

2. Put the flowers into a steamer basket and add a cup of water in the pressure cooker. Put the steamer basket with the carrots into the pan, seal the lid in place and cook the carrots for 4 about minutes at low pressure.

3. Quick release pressure and remove the steamer basket.

4. Transfer the carrots into a serving dish and serve the flowers. Season them with salt and drizzle some olive oil.

## 35: Spinach Artichoke Dip

*Serves: 4-6*

## Ingredients

Pinch of cayenne pepper

¼ teaspoon of black pepper, fresh ground

¼ teaspoon of garlic salt

½ cup of sour cream

1 cup of mozzarella cheese, shredded

1 cup of grated Parmesan cheese

1 cup of light mayonnaise

14 ounce can of artichoke hearts, drained and chopped

10 ounces of frozen spinach, chopped and thawed

## Directions

Combine all the ingredients, spoon into a lightly greased baking dish, and then tightly cover with foil. Now make a foil string to lift the baking dish.

Into the cooker, pour 2 cups of water and position the rack in the bottom.

Center the baking dish containing the contents and the foil strip and lower into the rack. Ensure that strip is well folded for it not to interfere with closing the lid.

Lock the lid in place and cook for 10 minutes at high pressure. Then turn off the pressure cooker, release the pressure and wait for the valve to drop.

Remove the lid and inspect whether the cheese is melted or pipping hot. You can then serve with tortilla chips or pita wedges.

# Section 5: Dessert Recipes

**36: Instant Pot Banoffee Pie**

**Serves: 8**

*Ingredients*

½ teaspoon vanilla essence

300ml Greek yoghurt

80g butter

1 can condensed milk

200g Digestive Biscuits

3 small bananas

Optional: Caramel Sauce

## Directions

Remove the labels off your condensed milk and lay it on its side at the bottom of your instant pot. Fill the pot with water until the whole can is covered by water.

Place the pot on manual for 35 minutes and ensure to set the valve on sealing.

As the milk cooks, add the butter to a saucepan and melt it, and then crush the digestive biscuits.

Once the butter melts, add the biscuits and mix well then place them at the bottom of the baking tin. Put in the fridge to cool and set.

After the time elapses, remove the milk carefully from the pot and leave it on your chopping board for 30 minutes to cool.

When cooled, pour the contents into a mixing bowl and slice the bananas into it and mix well.

Remove the crust from the fridge and add it to the ingredients in the mixing bowl at the base.

Just before you serve, mix together the yogurt and vanilla and pour it onto the Banoffee pie.

Optional: Drizzle some caramel sauce on top.

## 37: Crème Brûlée in the Pressure Cooker

*Serves: 6*

### Ingredients

8 egg yolks

1/3  cup of granulated sugar

pinch of salt

2 cups of heavy cream

1½ teaspoons of vanilla

6 tablespoons of superfine sugar

## Directions

Add 1½ cups of liquid to the cooking pot of an Instant Pot. Then put the trivet in the bottom.

Whisk together 1/3 cup of granulated sugar, egg yolks, and salt. Add inn vanilla and cream and whisk to incorporate. Use a pitcher or spout to strain the mixture into a measuring bowl; distribute the batter among 6 custard cups and cover using a foil.

Put the custard cups on the trivet of your Instant Pot. Stack the cups in a another layer, preferably using a second trivet between layers.

Lock the lid and cook for 6 minutes on high pressure. After the beep sounds, turn of the Instant Pot and natural release pressure for 10 minutes.

Open the lid and remove the custard cups, uncover them, and set to a wire rack to cool down. Once cool, keep refrigerated while covered with plastic wrap for 2 hours and up to 2 days.

To serve, sprinkle a tablespoon of sugar to cover each custard. To melt the sugar and form a crispy caramelized surface, move the flame of the torch above each custard in a circular motion.

## 38: Cheesecake with Shortbread Cookie Crust

***Serves: 8***

**Ingredients**

**For Crust**

2 tablespoons of butter, melted

1/3 cup of pecans, chopped

6 crushed shortbread toffee cookies

**For Filling**

3 eggs at room temperature

2 tablespoons of all-purpose flour

2 teaspoons of vanilla extract

1/3 cup of sour cream

1/3 cup of heavy cream

¾ cup of sugar

2 8-ounce packages of cream cheese

## Directions

Grease a 7-inch spring-form with non-stick cooking spray.

Combine the butter, chopped pecans, and cookies in a bowl. Bread evenly and then keep refrigerated for around 10 minutes.

Combine the sugar and cream cheese in a mixing bowl placed on medium high heat until smooth. Then blend in the floor, vanilla, heavy cream, and the sour cream.

Now mix the eggs one at a time to incorporate; follow this with the batter onto the prepared crust.

Position the trivet in the bottom of the cooker, add in a cup of water and then drop the pan using a sling into the trivet. To make a sling, just fold an 18-20 inch aluminum foil into 3 times lengthwise.

At this point, lock the lid in place and cook for 30 minutes at high pressure. Once done, natural release pressure for 10 minutes.

Allow to cool for 1-2 hours and then keep in the fridge for at least 2-3 hours or alternatively keep it overnight.

Serve topped with toffee bits, caramel ice cream topping, grated chocolate, or chopped pecans if you like.

## 39: Pressure Cooker Key Lime Pie

*Serves: 6-8*

## Ingredients

1 tablespoon of sugar

3 tablespoons of unsalted butter, melted

¾ cup of graham-cracker crumbs

## For filling

2 tablespoons of key lime zest, grated

1/3 cup of sour cream

½ cup of fresh key lime juice

4 large egg yolks

1 14-ounce can of condensed milk, sweetened

## Directions

Using non-stick spray, coat a 7-inch spring form pan and set it aside.

Mix the sugar, cracker crumbs, and butter in a small bowl. Press the mixture evenly in the bottom and up the sides of the pan.

Freeze for around 10 minutes.

Prepare the filling by beating the eggs in a large mixing bowl until light yellow.

Beat in condensed milk, blend until thickened, then add lime juice and continue to beat until smooth.

Now pour the batter in the pan on top of the crush and cover using aluminum foil.

Add a cup of water into an Instant Pot and put the trivet in the bottom. On a foil sling, carefully lower the filled pan into the center of the cooking pot.

Lock the lid and set the timer to 15 minutes. Cook on high pressure then turn off the cooker when time elapses. Natural release pressure for 10 minutes then do a quick release. Carefully open the lid and see if the middle is set. Cook for another 5 minutes if not yet done.

Remove the pan to a wire rack, uncover the aluminum foil, and allow time for the pie to cool and refrigerate for at least 4 hours while covered with plastic wrap.

Serve topped with whipped cream if you like.

## 40: Instant Pot Christmas Pudding

***Serves: 8***

## Ingredients

1 tablespoon of treacle

1 medium carrot finely grated

70g of self-rising flour

2 large eggs

70g of fresh breadcrumbs

1 teaspoon zest of a lemon

1 teaspoon of mixed spice

75g of dark muscovado sugar

75g of soft butter

4 balls of Stem Ginger, finely chopped

90ml of hazelnut liqueur

50g of finely chopped pecans

50g of finely chopped dried dates

200g of dried fruit

## Directions

First, soak the dried fruit in the liquor in a covered bowl overnight.

In a bowl, beat sugar and butter until light and fluffy then add the rest of the ingredients. Stir to blend.

Scrape the mixture into a buttered pudding basin and cover using an oiled or buttered grease-proof paper and a foil too. Fasten the paper and foil using a string or electric band beneath the lip of the basin.

Carefully lower the pudding basin onto the trivet and pour boiling water to just below the level of the foil.

Lock the lid in place and set the timer to 10 minutes. Cook under high pressure until the beep sounds then quick release pressure.

Set to low pressure and cook for 45 minutes then do a quick release. Open the lid and remove the pudding onto a rack to cool.

Remove the paper and foil and replace with fresh ones. Allow to cool and darken until ready to cook.

To cook, put the pudding on a trivet and pour boiling water. Set the timer to 20 minutes then natural release pressure.

Invert into a serving platter and portion it. Serve with rum, rum sauce, custard, or brandy butter if you like.

## 41: Pears Stewed in Red Wine

***Serves: 4***

## Ingredients

4 tablespoons heavy cream

1 cup frozen raspberries

3/4 cup red wine

4 firm pears, peeled with stems on

1/4 teaspoon mace

2 cinnamon sticks

2 slices lemon

1/2 cup sugar

2 cups water

## Directions

1. Mix together mace, cinnamon sticks, lemon, sugar and water in the pressure cooker and simmer to dissolve the sugar.

2. Add the pears into a steamer basket then lower into the pressure cooker. Lock the lid and cook for 2 minutes on high pressure.

3. Quick release pressure and open the lid. Now add in red wine.

4. Lock the lid and cook for another 2 minutes then quick release. Lift out the steamer basket and move the pears to a deep container.

5. Boil the sauce until syrupy, and then pour over the pears.

6. To serve, puree raspberries in a blender, then spoon 4 tablespoons of the puree onto serving bowls.

7. Put a pear in each dish, then spoon the pureed raspberries over the pears. Drizzle the sauce onto the pears. Dribble a tablespoon of cream over the sauce and swirl the cream into the sauce using a knife to make a creative design. Serve and enjoy!

## 42: Instant Pot Custard

***Serves 4***

### Ingredients

1 cup water

1/2 teaspoon vanilla extract

1/3 cup sugar

2 eggs

2 cups milk

### Directions

1. Scald the milk then let it cool. Mix together sugar and the eggs, then add in the milk. Continue to stir and then add in the vanilla extract.

2. Pour the mixture into custard cups and use aluminum foil to cover.

3. Add sufficient water to the pressure cooker and then position the trivet and steamer basket in the cooker.

4. Put the foil-covered custard cups into the steamer basket, and lock the cooker in place.

5. Bring the pressure cooker to pressure and cook for 3 minutes at high pressure.

6. Quick release, and remove the lid. Cool the custard before serving.

# I need your help...

We have come to the end of the book. Thank you for reading and congratulations for reading until the end.

I hope you have learnt a lot on how to unleash the full power of your Instant Pot by making delicious recipes.

If you found the book valuable, can you recommend it to others? One way to do that is to post a review on Amazon.

Finally, if you enjoyed this book, then I'd like to ask you for a favor, would you be kind enough to leave a review for this book on Amazon? It'd be greatly appreciated!

I want to reach as many people as I can with this book, and more reviews will help me accomplish that!

If you have any questions or problems, please contact us: hello@freedomdestination.com

Thank you and good luck!

# Preview Of 'Dash Diet: Cookbook For Weight Loss With Action Plan And Easy Recipes'

## What Is The DASH Diet?

The DASH (Dietary Approaches to Stop Hypertension) diet is an eating plan especially recommended for those with pre-hypertension or hypertension (high blood pressure). This diet helps in lowering blood pressure by availing key nutrients such as magnesium, calcium, and potassium all of which are associated with lower blood pressure. The DASH diet is rich in vegetables, fruits, nonfat dairy or low fat. It also includes lean meats, poultry and fish, whole grains, beans and nuts.

While the DASH diet was initially developed to help lower blood pressure, it is now also considered quite effective in weight loss, promoting hearth health, lowering inflammation and cholesterol.

Let us learn more about how this diet can do all the above:

## Weight Loss

To lose weight, you have to create a calorie deficit. The DASH diet does not stress on calorie reduction; however, it recommends consumption of whole grains, vegetables, fruits and lean meats. Whole grains, fruits and vegetables are high in fiber, which is quite filling but relatively lower in calories. Meat, poultry, and fish being protein take quite some time to be digested; hence, you feel fuller for longer. If you combine this and reduce your intake of processed sugars, sweets and unhealthy fats, you will create a caloric deficit without too much work, which will lead to weight loss.

The great thing is that you will not feel hungry even as you lose weight because all the foods you will be eating are quite filling.

## Lowers Blood Pressure

The DASH diet helps in lowering blood pressure due to its food composition. The DASH diet is rich in fiber, calcium, magnesium, and potassium; and has a low content of saturated fat and sodium. Adding more of these nutrients to your diet improves the electrolyte balance in your body thus allowing it to excrete the excess fluid that contributes to high blood pressure. These nutrients also reduce blood pressure by promoting the relaxation of blood vessels. Most people suffering from high blood pressure usually have these nutrients in deficiency so the DASH diet is quite effective at providing these nutrients; thus, lowering blood pressure.

## Lower Cholesterol Levels

The DASH diet recommends intake of whole grains, which are high in fiber. Oats, brown rice, and whole-wheat products are excellent sources of fiber. Adequate fiber in your body has been shown to reduce cholesterol levels. Women should obtain 25 grams of fiber per day while men should aim for 38 grams.

## Manages Insulin Resistance

The DASH is further favorable for those people with insulin resistance, pre-diabetes or diabetes as it helps in improving insulin sensitivity. The combination of nutrients and foods in the DASH diet may have an effect on various cellular targets that ultimately elevates changes in your body composition during weight loss thus effecting favorable impact on insulin action.

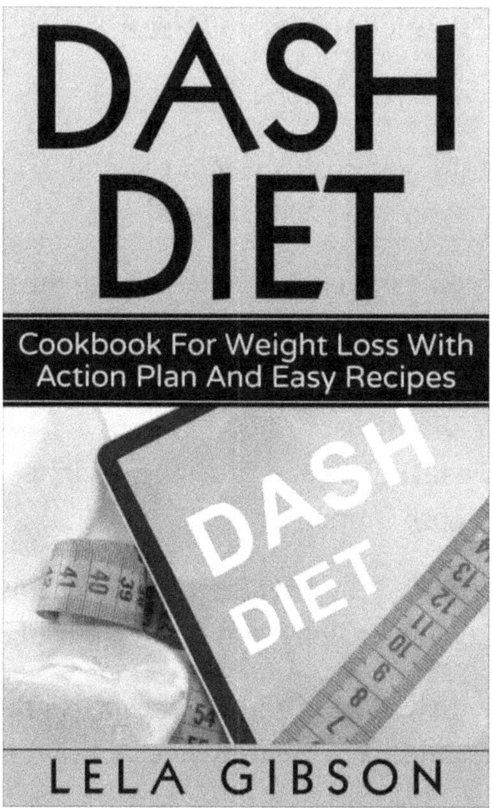


Check out the rest of Dash Diet: Cookbook For Weight Loss With Action Plan And Easy Recipes on Amazon, go to http://amzn.to/2mPW21b

# Check Out My Other Books

Below you'll find some of my other popular books that are popular on Amazon and Kindle as well.

Alternatively, you can visit my author page on Amazon to see other work done by me.

20 Easy And Fast Diet Tips For Losing Weight – An Easy-To-Follow Weight Loss Guide

Belly Diet: The Zero Belly Diet Step-By-Step Guide Which Will Help You To Lose Your Belly And Enjoy Your Flat Belly

Anti-Inflammatory Diet Guide – The Guide To Reduce Inflammation And Live A Healthy Life Without Pain

Dash Diet: Cookbook For Weight Loss With Action Plan And Easy Recipes

Clean Eating: Cookbook And Guide To Restore Your Body's Natural Balance And Eat Healthy

Negative Calorie Diet: Cookbook & Guide Which Help You To Burn Body Fat, Lose Weight And Live Healthy

Smart Fat: Cookbook With Fat Meals Which Help You To Lose Weight, Get Healthy And Improve Brain Function

Freedom: How To Make Money Online And Become Financially Free By Creating Passive Income

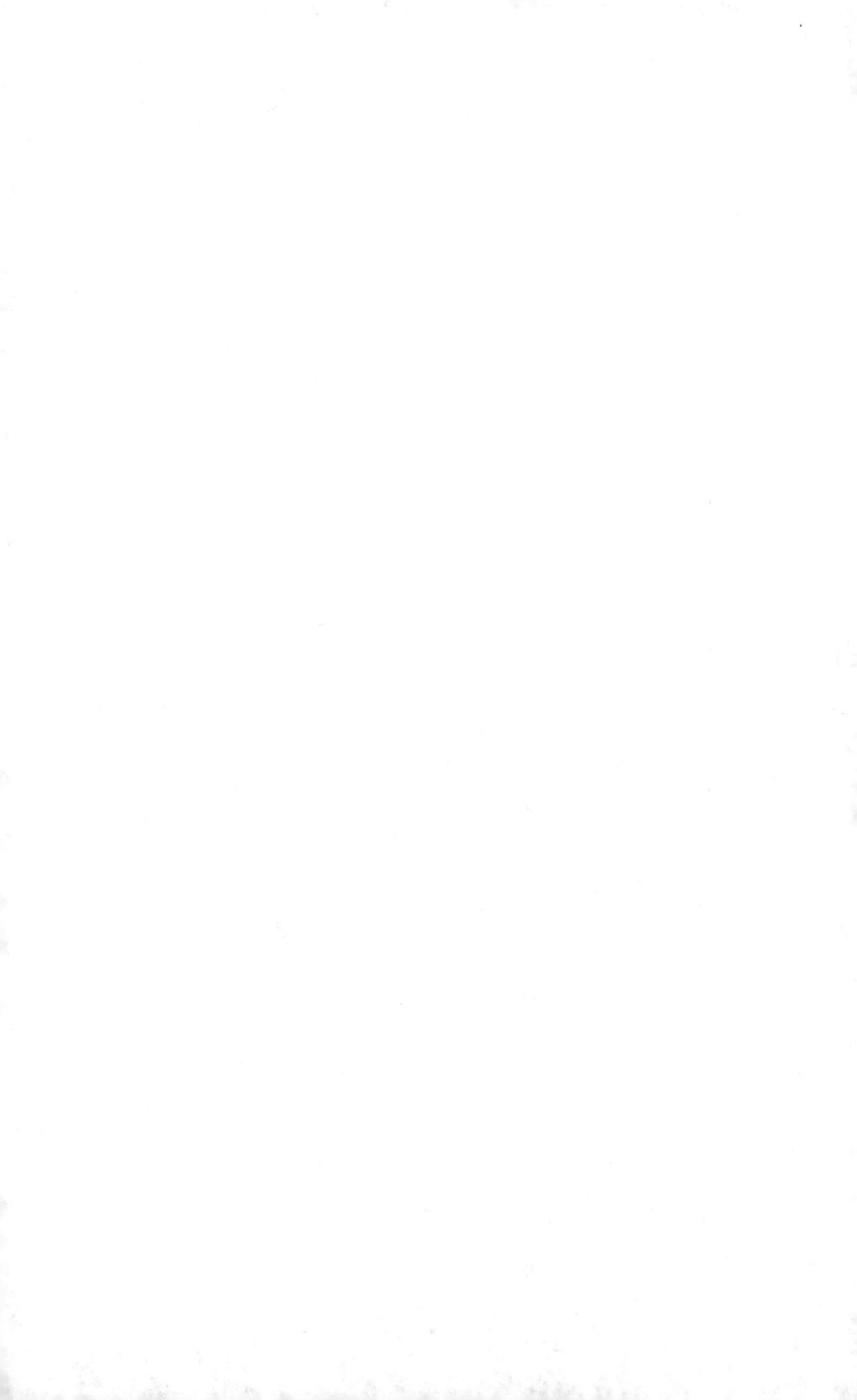